The Best Sirtfood Cookbook

An Easy-To-Follow Recipes to Shed Fat and also Enjoy Your Life

by Ursula Matin

Sommario

Introduction

In time, the Sirtfood diet regimen has actually drawn in lots of VIPs from the globe of enjoyment and also national politics due to its simpleness as well as performance without needing massive sacrifices.

It is based upon consuming the "ideal" food, that makes certain to trigger the sirtuins, the supposed slimness genetics in each people.

The intake of such foods sees to it to shed 3 kg each week without depriving the body or polluting it with incorrect foods.

I advise speaking with a physician to make a diet regimen strategy and also to obtain suggestions for light exercise.

Chapter 1 Breakfast Recipes

Soy and Zucchini Omelette

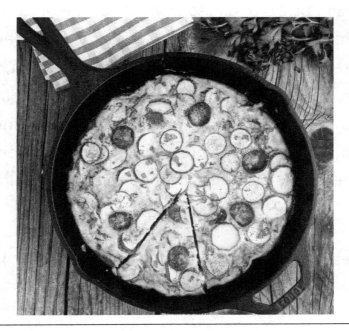

Preparation time: 10 minutes
Cooking time: 10 minutes
Servings: 2

Ingredients: 2 teaspoons of olive oil

2 small zucchini (100 g) 3 teaspoons of flour 00 (40 g)

2 pinches of salt 1/3 third glass of soy milk (60 g)

Directions: Cut the zucchini into very thin slices (with a greater with the appropriate blade, or with a potato peeler, not with a knife). Put the flour and salt in a soup plate, add the soy milk a little at a time and 2 fingers of water, and stir quickly with a fork so as not to form lumps. You have to get a batter that's not too dense, quite liquid. Pour in the zucchini slices and stir well. In a non-stick frying pan put 2 s of oil (so as to cover the bottom just barely) and heat over a high heat. When the oil is hot, pour the batter and level well with a wooden spatula. Put the lid on it and leave the fire high, then after about half a minute lower the fire a little. The omelette must cook in all about 10 minutes, and in this time should be turned a couple of times, so that both sides are browned (you can cut it into 4 slices and turn them one at a time). Hold the lid for the first 5 minutes, for the remaining 5 minutes let it brown without the lid.

Nutrition: Calories: 115 Net carbs: 24.4g Fat: 0.6g Fiber: 4.6g Protein: 5.6g

Kale Omelette

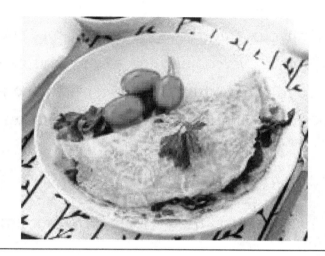

Preparation time: 5 minutes
Cooking time: 5 minutes
Servings: 1

Ingredients:

Eggs – 3 Garlic – 1 small glove Kale – 2 handfuls

Goat cheese or any cheese of your choice Sliced onion – ¼ cup

Extra virgin olive oil – 2 teaspoons

Directions:

Mince the garlic, and finely shred the kale. Break the eggs into a bowl, add a pinch of salt. Beat until well combined. Place a pan to heat over medium heat. Add one teaspoon of olive oil, add the onion and kale, cook for approx. Five minutes, or until the onion has softened and the kale is wilted. Add the garlic and cook for another two minutes.

Add one teaspoon of olive oil into the egg mixture, mix and add into the pan. Use your spatula to move the cooked egg toward the center and move the pan so that the uncooked egg mixture goes towards the edges. Add the cheese into the pan just before the egg is fully cooked, then leave for a minute.

Nutrition:

Calories: 38 Net carbs: 7.9g Fat: 0.2g Fiber: 2.9g Protein: 2.5g

Turmeric Scrambled Eggs

Preparation time: 10 minutes
Cooking time: 10 minutes
Servings: 3

Ingredients:

Butter - 1 tablespoon Large spinach – 1 handful Large eggs – 6

Salt & pepper to taste Turmeric powder - 2 teaspoons

Large tomato – 1 (chopped) Coconut oil - 1 teaspoon

Directions:

Break the eggs into a medium bowl, whisk and add the pepper, salt, and turmeric. Mix together and set aside. Heat the coconut oil in a small fry pan, add the chopped tomato and cook for about 2 to 3 minutes, until soft. Add the spinach into the pan and cook for another two minutes. Set aside. Add the butter into a small nonstick saucepan to melt under medium-low heat, then add the egg mixture. Use your spatula to push the eggs from side to side across the pan.

Add the tomato and spinach to the pan when the eggs are almost done.

Once the egg is cooked, serve immediately.

Nutrition:

Calories: 308 Net carbs: 16.8g Fat: 12.9g Fiber: 1.7g Protein: 20.9g

Gluten Omelette

Preparation time: 1 hour 25 minutes
Cooking time: 6 minutes
Servings: 2

Ingredients: 1 kg of flour Olive oil

2 pinches of vegetable cube

A handful of parsley A few drops of lemon

Half a of salt

Directions: First we have to get the gluten, then we put the flour in a container and knead it with water as if we wanted to make bread. Let the dough rest for about an hour. After the resting period, we take our loaf of bread, tear off a piece not too big and wash it under water until only the gluten remains in our hands (the rinse water must remain almost transparent, no longer white as at the beginning); we repeat the operation for the rest of the pasta. Having finally obtained our gluten, iron it with our hands until it forms a medallion about one cm thick, put it in a pot, cover it with water (not too much, just enough to cover it), add half a of salt and boil it for 6 minutes, being careful not to stick it on the bottom and turn it on the other side halfway through cooking. We take our gluten out of the water and squeeze it with a fork to make it lose the excess liquid, pour the olive oil into a large pan and fry the gluten. While frying, we put a pinch of dice on both sides, chopped parsley and a few drops of lemon. As soon as it's golden and crisp it'll be ready. Place it on blotting paper and serve with a few drops of lemon and a nice salad.

Nutrition: Calories: 381 Net carbs: 4.6g Fat: 11.8g Fiber: 0.5g Protein: 34.4g

Tomato and Mushroom Omelette

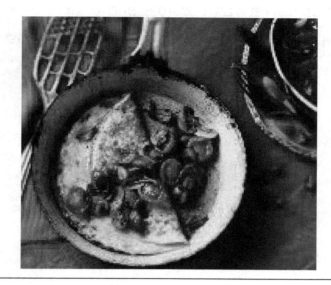

Preparation time: 10 minutes
Cooking time: 15 minutes
Servings: 2

Ingredients:

4 teaspoons of chickpea flour 5 medium tomatoes

One medium onion one Can of mushrooms Baking powder one

Glass of water 1/4 of lemon oil for frying to taste

Directions:

Thinly slice the onion and fry it for 5 minutes, then add the chopped tomatoes and drained mushrooms; let it run on medium heat until the water that the tomatoes will tend to release has dried. In a plate, mix the chickpea flour with baking powder, a pinch of salt, a splash of lemon and a glass of water. Make sure the mixture is as velvety as possible and pour it into the pan. Fry for 5 minutes stirring continuously. Dust with a spoonful of yeast and serve.

Nutrition:

Calories: 173 Net carbs: 5.8g Fat: 3.2g Fiber: 1g Protein: 8g

Parsley Smoothie

Preparation time: 2 minutes
Cooking time: 2 minutes
Servings: 2

Ingredients:

Flat-leaf parsley - 1 cup Juice of two lemons Apple – 1 (core removed)

Avocado – 1 Chopped kale - 1 cup Peeled fresh ginger – 1 knob

Honey - 1 tablespoon Iced water - 2 cups

Directions:

Add all the ingredients except the avocado into your blender. Blend on high until smooth, then add the avocado, then set your blender to slow speed and blend until creamy. Add a little more iced water if the smoothie is too thick.

Nutrition:

Calories: 5

Net carbs: 1.1g

Fiber: 0.2g

Protein: 0.2g

Matcha Overnight Oats

Preparation time: 12 hours
Cooking time: 0 minutes
Servings: 2

Ingredients:

For the Oats

Chia seeds - 2 teaspoon Rolled oats – 3 oz.

Matcha powder - 1 teaspoon

Honey - 1 teaspoon

Almond milk – 1 ½ cups

Ground cinnamon - 2 pinches

For the Topping

Apple – 1 (peeled, cored and chopped)

A handful of mixed nuts

Pumpkin seeds – 1 teaspoon

Directions:

Get your oats ready a night before. Place the chia seeds and the oats in a container or bowl. In a different jug or bowl, add the matcha powder and one tablespoon of almond milk and whisk with a hand-held mixer until you get a smooth paste, then add the rest of the milk and mix thoroughly. Pour the milk mixture over the oats, add the honey and cinnamon, and then stir well. Cover the bowl with a lid and place in the fridge overnight. When you want to eat, transfer the oats to two serving bowls, then top with the nuts, pumpkin seeds, and chopped apple.

Nutrition: Calories: 20 Net carbs: 4.1g Fat: 0.2g Fiber: 1.4g Protein: 1.5g

Dark Chocolate Protein Truffles

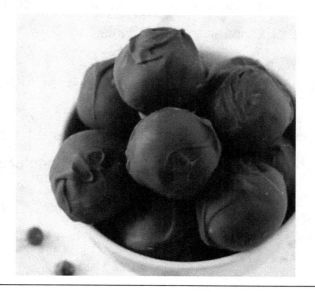

Preparation time: 10 minutes
Cooking time: 10 minutes
Servings: 8

Ingredients:

Coconut oil - ¼ cup Vanilla whey protein powder - ¼ cup

Medjool dates - ¼ cup (chopped) Almond milk - ¼ cup

Honey - 2 tablespoon Steel-cut oats - ⅛ cup

Coconut flour - 1 tablespoon

Dark chocolate bars, minimum 85% cacao – 2

Directions:

Mix the protein powder, honey, almond milk, dates, coconut flour, and oats in a bowl, then mold the mixture into eight balls.

Melt the coconut oil and chocolate over medium heat in a pot.

Turn off the heat once melted and allow the chocolate to cool for about five to ten minutes. Dip each of the balls into the melted chocolate until well covered.

Place the balls in the freezer to harden.

Nutrition:

Calories: 240 Net carbs: 20g Total fat: 10g

Refreshing Watermelon Juice

Preparation time: 2 minutes
Cooking time: 0 minutes
Servings: 1

Ingredients:

Young kale leaves - 20g (stalks removed)

Cucumber – ½ (peeled, seeds removed and roughly chopped)

Watermelon chunks - 250g

Mint leaves - 250g

Directions:

Add all the ingredients into your blender or juicer. Blend and enjoy.

Nutrition:

Calories: 71

Net carbs: 17.9g

Fat: 0.3g

Fiber: 1g

Protein: 1.4g

Matcha Granola with Berries

Preparation Time: 5 minutes
Cooking time: 20 minutes
Servings: 4

Ingredients: Rolled oats - 1 cup

Coconut oil- 2 tablespoon

Mixed nuts - ½ cup (chopped)

Pumpkin seeds - 1 tablespoon

Matcha powder - 1 tablespoon

Strawberries - 1 cup (halved or quartered)

Sesame seeds - 1 tablespoon

Ground cinnamon - ½ teaspoon

Runny honey - 3 tablespoons

Blueberries - 2/3 cup

Greek yogurt - 1 ¾ cups

Directions:

Heat your oven to 325 degrees F. place parchment paper on a baking tray.

Heat the coconut oil under low heat until it melts. Put off the heat and stir in the seeds, nuts, and oats. Add the cinnamon, matcha powder, and honey, then mix thoroughly.

Evenly spread the granola mixture over the lined baking tray and place in the oven to bake for about fifteen minutes, until crisp and toasted – turn it 2 to 3 times.

Remove from the oven to cool, then store in an airtight container.

To serve, layer the yogurt in the serving dishes, then add the berries and granola.

Nutrition:

Calories: 133

Net carbs: 18.6g

Fat: 5.8g

Fiber: 1g

Protein: 1.9g

Coffee and Cashew Smoothie

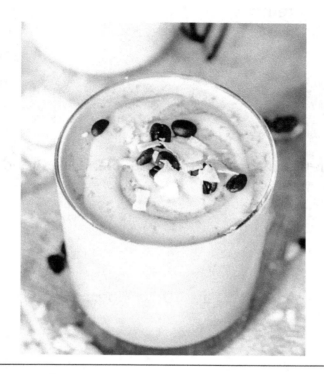

Preparation Time: 5 minutes
Cooking time: 0 minutes
Servings: 1

Ingredients:

Cashew butter - 1 teaspoon

Chilled cashew - ½ glass

Tahini - 1 teaspoon

Medjool date – 1 (pitted and chopped)

Espresso coffee - 1 shot

Ground cinnamon - ½ teaspoon

Tiny pinch of salt

Directions:

Add all the ingredients into a high-speed blender. Blend until creamy and smooth.

Nutrition:

Calories: 360 Net carbs: 33.1g Fat: 19.7g Fiber: 5.3g Protein: 14.1g

Buckwheat Pita Bread Sirtfood

Preparation time: 20 minutes
Cooking time: 30 minutes
Servings: 6

Ingredients: Sea salt - 1 teaspoon Polenta for dusting

Packet dried yeast - 1 x 8 gram Lukewarm water - 375ml

Extra virgin olive oil - 3 tablespoon Buckwheat flour - 500 grams

Directions:

Add the yeast in the lukewarm water, mix and set aside for about 10 to 15 minutes to activate. Mix the buckwheat flour, olive oil, salt, and yeast mixture. Work slowly to make a dough. Cover and place in a warm spot for approx. one hour – this is to get the dough to rise. Divide the dough into six parts. Shape one of the pieces into a flat disc and place between two sheets of a baking paper. Gently roll out the dough into a round pita shape that is approximately ¼-inch thick. Use a fork to pierce the dough a few times, then dust lightly with polenta. Heat up your cast iron pan and brush the pan with olive oil. Cook the pita for about 5 minutes on one side, until puffy, then turn to the other side and repeat. Fill the pita with your preferred veggies and meat, then serve immediately.

Nutrition:

Calories: 124 Net carbs: 25g Fat: 0.5g Fiber: 1g Protein: 4.1g

No-Bake Apple Crisp Recipe

Preparation time: 10 minutes
Cooking time: 0 minutes
Servings: 8

Ingredients: Apples - 8 (peeled, cored and chopped)

Cinnamon - 2 teaspoons (divided) Raisins - 1 cup (soaked and drained)

Lemon juice - 2 tablespoons Medjool dates - 1 cup Walnuts - 2 cups

Sea salt - ⅛ teaspoon Nutmeg - ¼ teaspoon

Directions:

Add one teaspoon of cinnamon, the raisins, two apples, and the nutmeg into your food processor. Process until smooth. Toss the remaining chopped apples and the lemon juice in a big bowl. Pour the apple puree over the apples in the bowl and mix well. Transfer the mixture into a medium-sized baking dish and keep aside. Add the remaining cinnamon, dates, sea salt, and walnuts into your food processor. Pulse until coarsely grounded. Do not over mix. Sprinkle the mixture over the apples and use your hands to press down lightly. Allow to sit for a few hours for the flavor to marinate or serve immediately.

Nutrition:

Calories: 243 Net carbs: 22g Fat: 8.6g Fiber: 0.5g Protein: 19g

Matcha Latte

Preparation time: 2 minutes
Cooking time: 3 minutes
Servings: 1

Ingredients:

Unsweetened rice milk - 1 mug

Date syrup – ½ teaspoon (optional)

Matcha powder - 1 teaspoon

Directions:

Heat the matcha and milk in a pan and froth it until it gets hot, stir in your preferred sweetener.

Pour into your cup and Enjoy!

Nutrition:

Calories: 205Net carbs: 42.4g

Fat: 2.5g Fiber: 0.5g Protein: 2.8g

Melon and Grape Juice

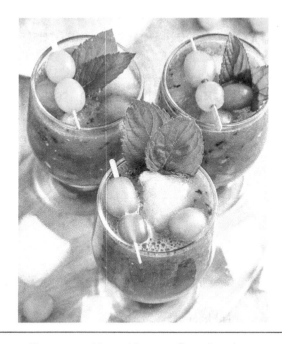

Preparation time: 2 minutes
Cooking time: 0 minutes
Servings: 1

Ingredients:

Red seedless grapes – 1 cup

Young spinach leaves – 1 ounce (stalks removed)

Cucumber – ½ (peel if you like, halved, seeds removed and chopped roughly)

Cantaloupe melon – 1 cup (peeled, deseeded and chopped into chunks)

Directions:

Add all the ingredients into your juicer and blend until smooth.

Nutrition:

Calories: 125 Net carbs: 7g Fat: 0.1g

Protein: 0.6g

Blackcurrant and Kale Smoothie

Preparation Time: 3 minutes
Cooking time: 0 minutes
Servings: 2

Ingredients:

Ripe banana – 1

Honey - 2 teaspoon

Baby kale leaves - 10 (stalks removed)

Freshly made green tea - 1 cup

Blackcurrants – 1/3 cup (washed and stalks removed)

Ice cubes – 6

Directions:

Add the honey into the warm green tea. Stir until dissolved.

Add all the ingredients into your blender. Blend until smooth.

Serve immediately.

Nutrition: Calories: 18

Net carbs: 4.3g Fat: 0.1g Protein: 0.4g

Chapter 2 Lunch Recipes

Pesto Green Beans

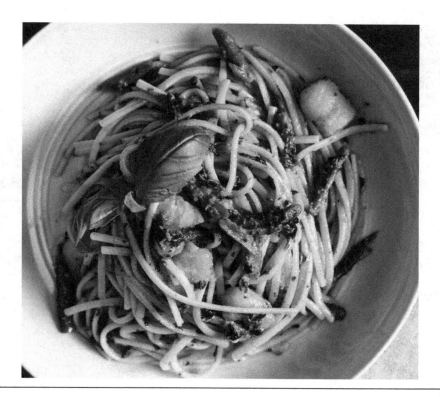

Preparation time: 10 minutes
Cooking time: 15 minutes
Servings: 4

Ingredients:

2 tablespoons olive oil

2 tablespoon sweet paprika

Juice of 1 lemon

2 tablespoons basil pesto

1 lb. trimmed and halved green beans

¼ tablespoon black pepper

1 sliced red onion

Directions:

Heat up a pan with the oil over medium-high heat, add the onion, stir and sauté for 5 minutes.

Add the beans and the rest of the ingredients, toss, cook over medium heat for 10 minutes, divide between plates and serve.

Nutrition:

Calories: 280

Fat: 10g

Carbs: 13.9g

Protein: 4.7g

Sugars: 0.8g

Sodium: 138mg

Spinach Salad with Green Asparagus and Salmon

Preparation time: 10 minutes
Cooking time: 0 minutes
Servings: 2

Ingredients:

2 hands Spinach

2 pieces Egg

120 g smoked salmon

100 g Asparagus tips

150 g Cherry tomatoes

Lemon 1 / 2 pieces

1 teaspoon Olive oil

Directions:

Cook the eggs the way you like them.

Heat a pan with a little oil and fry the asparagus.

Halve cherry tomatoes.

Place the spinach on a plate and spread the asparagus tips, cherry tomatoes and smoked salmon on top.

Scare, peel and halve the eggs. Add them to the salad.

Squeeze the lemon over the lettuce and drizzle some olive oil over it.

Season the salad with a little salt and pepper.

Nutrition:

Calories: 107 Fat: 4.8g Net Carbs: 11.2g

Fiber: 1.4g Protein: 5.1g

Brunoised Salad

Preparation time: 10 minutes
Cooking time: 0 minutes
Servings: 3

Ingredients:

1 piece Meat tomato

1 / 2 pieces Zucchini

1 / 2 pieces Red bell pepper

1 / 2 pieces yellow bell pepper

1 / 2 pieces Red onion

3 sprigs fresh parsley

1 / 4 pieces Lemon

2 tablespoons Olive oil

Directions:

Finely dice the tomatoes, zucchini, peppers and red onions to get a brunoise.

Mix all the cubes in a bowl.

Chop parsley and mix in the salad.

Squeeze the lemon over the salad and add the olive oil.

Season with salt and pepper.

Nutrition:

Calories: 170

Fat: 3.6g

Net Carbs: 8.7g

Fiber: 2g

Protein: 1.5g

Buns with Chicken and Cucumber

| Preparation time: 15 minutes |
| Cooking time: 0 minutes |
| Servings: 4 |

Ingredients:

12 slices Chicken Breast (Spread)

1 piece Cucumber

1 piece Red pepper

50g fresh basil

3 tablespoons Olive oil

3 tablespoons Pine nuts

Garlic 1 clove

Directions:

Wash the cucumber and cut into thin strips, then cut the peppers into thin strips.

Put the basil, olive oil, pine nuts and garlic in a food processor. Stir to an even pesto.

Season the pesto and season with salt and pepper if necessary.

Place a slice of chicken fillet on a plate, brush with 1 teaspoon of pesto and top the strips with cucumber and peppers.

Carefully roll up the chicken fillet to create a nice roll.

If necessary, secure the rolls with a cocktail skewer.

Nutrition:

Calories: 90 Fat: 8g Protein: 4g

Hazelnut Balls

Preparation time: 40 minutes
Cooking time: 0 minutes
Servings: 1

Ingredients:

130g Dates

140g Hazelnuts

2 tablespoon Cocoa powder

1 / 2 teaspoon Vanilla extract

1 teaspoon Honey

Directions:

Put the hazelnuts in a food processor and grind them until you get hazelnut flour (of course you can also use ready-made hazelnut flour).

Put the hazelnut flour in a bowl and set aside.

Put the dates in the food processor and grind them until you get a ball.

Add the hazelnut flour, vanilla extract, cocoa and honey and pulse until you get a nice and even mix.

Remove the mixture from the food processor and turn it into beautiful balls.

Store the balls in the fridge.

Nutrition:

Calories: 722

Fat: 69.8g Net Carbs: 19.2g

Fiber: 11.2g Protein: 17.1g

Stuffed Eggplants

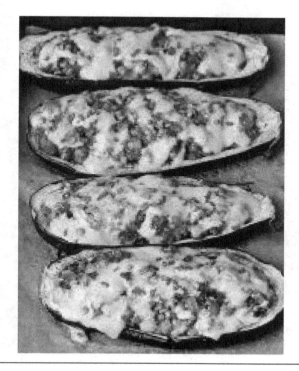

Preparation time: 10 minutes
Cooking time: 30 minutes
Servings: 2

Ingredients:

4 pieces Eggplant

3 tablespoons Coconut oil

1 piece Onion

250g Ground beef

2 cloves Garlic

3 pieces Tomatoes

1 tablespoon Tomato paste

1 hand Capers

1 hand fresh basil

Directions:

Finely chop the onion and garlic. Cut the tomatoes into cubes and shred the basil leaves.

Bring a large pot of water to a boil, add the eggplants and let it cook for about 5 minutes.

Drain, let cool slightly and remove the pulp with a spoon (leave a rim about 1 cm thick around the skin). Cut the pulp finely and set aside.

Put the eggplants in a baking dish.

Preheat the oven to 175 ° C.

Heat 3 tablespoons of coconut oil in a pan on a low flame and glaze the onion.

Add the minced meat and garlic and fry until the beef is loose.

Add the finely chopped eggplants, tomato pieces, capers, and basil and tomato paste and fry them on the pan with the lid for 10 minutes.

Season with salt and pepper.

Fill the eggplant with the beef mixture and bake in the oven for about 20 minutes.

Nutrition:

Calories: 166

Fat: 3.8g

Net Carbs: 8.3g

Fiber: 2.4g

Protein: 0.8g

Chicken Teriyaki with Cauliflower Rice

Preparation time: 300 minutes
Cooking time: 40 minutes
Servings: 3

Ingredients:

500g Chicken breast

90ml Coconut aminos

2 tablespoons Coconut blossom sugar

1 tablespoon Olive oil

1 teaspoon Sesame oil

50g fresh ginger

2 cloves Garlic

250g Chinese cabbage

1 piece Leek

2 pieces Red peppers

1 piece Cauliflower (rice)

1 piece Onion

1 teaspoon Ghee

50g fresh coriander

1 piece Lime

Directions:

Cut the chicken into cubes. Mix coconut aminos, coconut blossom sugar, olive oil and sesame oil in a small bowl.

Finely chop the ginger and garlic and add to the marinade. Put the chicken in the marinade in the fridge overnight.

Roughly cut Chinese cabbage, leek, garlic and paprika and add to the slow cooker. Finally add the marinated chicken and let it cook for about 2 to 4 hours.

When the chicken is almost ready, you can cut the cauliflower into small florets. Then put the florets in a food processor and pulse briefly to prepare rice.

Finely chop an onion, heat a pan with a teaspoon of ghee and fry the onion. Then add the cauliflower rice and fry briefly.

Spread the chicken and cauliflower rice on the plates and garnish with a little chopped coriander and a wedge of lime.

Nutrition:

Calories: 506 Fat: 4.4g Net Carbs: 90.8g

Protein: 25.9g

Curry Chicken with Pumpkin Spaghetti

Preparation time: 5 minutes
Cooking time: 45 minutes
Servings: 5

Ingredients:

500 g Chicken breast

2 teaspoons Chili powder

1 piece Onion   1 clove Garlic

2 teaspoons Ghee

3 tablespoon Curry powder

500 ml Coconut milk (can)

200g Pineapple   200g Mango

1 piece Red pepper

1 piece Butternut squash

25 g Spring onion   25 g fresh coriander

Directions:

Cut the chicken into strips and season with pepper, salt and chili powder. Then put the chicken in the slow cooker.

Finely chop the onion and garlic and lightly fry with 2 teaspoons of ghee. Then add the curry powder.

Deglaze with the coconut milk after a minute. Add the sauce to the slow cooker along with the pineapple, mango cubes and chopped peppers and let it cook for 2 to 4 hours.

Cut the pumpkin into long pieces and make spaghetti out of it with a spiralizer (that's not easy, it works better with a carrot).

Briefly fry the pumpkin spaghetti in the pan and spread the chicken curry on top.

Garnish with thinly sliced spring onions and chopped coriander.

Nutrition:

Calories: 160Fat: 8.6gNet Carbs: 6.1g

Fiber: 1.2gProtein: 14.8g

French Style Chicken Thighs

Preparation time: 10 minutes
Cooking time: 4 hours
Servings: 6

Ingredients:

700 g Chicken leg 1 tablespoon Olive oil

2 pieces Onion 4 pieces Carrot

2 cloves Garlic 8 stems Celery

25g fresh rosemary 25g Fresh thyme

25 g fresh parsley

Directions:

Season the chicken with olive oil, pepper and salt and rub it into the meat.

Roughly cut onions, carrots, garlic and celery and add to the slow cooker. Place the chicken on top and finally sprinkle a few sprigs of rosemary, thyme and parsley on top. Let it cook for at least four hours.

Serve with a delicious salad, enjoy your meal!

Nutrition: Calories: 459 Fat: 34.8g

Net Carbs: 6.2g Fiber: 1.3g Protein: 29.7g

Spicy Ribs with Roasted Pumpkin

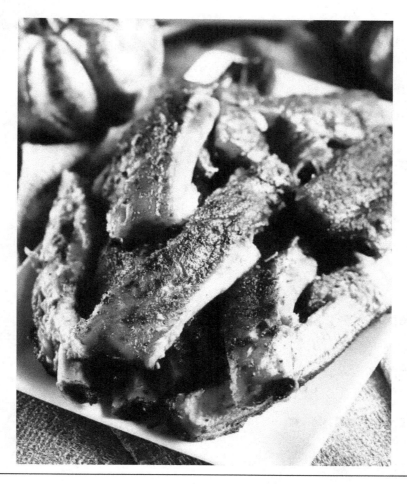

Preparation time: 24 hours
Cooking time: 4 hours
Servings: 3

Ingredients:

400 g Spare ribs

4 tablespoons Coconut-Aminos

2 tablespoons Honey

1 tablespoon Olive oil

50g Spring onions

Garlic 2 cloves

1 piece green chili peppers

1 piece Onion

1 piece Red pepper

1 piece Red pepper

For the roasted pumpkin:

Pumpkin 1 piece

Coconut oil 1 tablespoon

Paprika powder 1 tablespoon

Directions:

Marinate the ribs the day before.

Cut the ribs into pieces with four ribs each. Place the coconut aminos, honey and olive oil in a mixing bowl and mix. Chop the spring onions, garlic and green peppers and add them. Spread the ribs on plastic containers and pour the marinade over them. Leave them in the fridge overnight.

Cut the onions, peppers and peppers into pieces and put them in the slow cooker. Spread the ribs, including the marinade, and let them cook for at least 4 hours.

Preheat the oven to 200 ° C for the pumpkin.

Cut the pumpkin into moons and place on a baking sheet lined with parchment paper.

Spread a tablespoon of coconut oil on the baking sheet and season with paprika, pepper and salt. Roast the pumpkin in the oven for about 20 minutes and serve with the spare ribs.

Nutrition:

Calories: 65

Fat: 1.3g

Protein: 12.4 g

Roast Beef with Grilled Vegetables

Preparation time: 10 minutes
Cooking time: 30 minutes
Servings: 4

Ingredients:

500g Roast beef

1 clove Garlic (pressed)

1 teaspoon fresh rosemary

400g Broccoli

200g Carrot

400g Zucchini

4 tablespoons Olive oil

Directions:

Rub the roast beef with freshly ground pepper, salt, garlic and rosemary.

Heat a grill pan over high heat and grill the roast beef for about 20 minutes or until the meat shows nice brown marks on all sides.

Then wrap in aluminum foil and let it rest for a while.

Cut the roast beef into thin slices before serving.

Preheat the oven to 205 ° C. Put all the vegetables in a baking dish.

Drizzle the vegetables with a little olive oil and season with curry powder and / or chili flakes. Put in the oven and bake for 30 minutes or until the vegetables are done.

Nutrition:

Calories: 56

Fat: 3.6g

Protein: 5.4g

Vegan Thai Green Curry

Preparation time: 20 minutes
Cooking time: 4 hours 15 minutes
Servings: 2

Ingredients:

2 pieces green chilies 1 piece Onion

1 clove Garlic

1 teaspoon fresh ginger (grated)

25g fresh coriander

1 teaspoon Ground caraway

1 piece Lime (juice)

1 teaspoon Coconut oil

500 ml Coconut milk

1 piece Zucchini

1 piece Broccoli

1 piece Red pepper

For the cauliflower rice:

1 teaspoon Coconut oil

1 piece Cauliflower

Directions:

For cauliflower rice, cut the cauliflower into florets and place in the food processor. Pulse briefly until rice has formed. Put aside.

Cut the green peppers, onions, garlic, fresh ginger and coriander into large pieces and combine with the caraway seeds and the juice of 1 lime in a food processor or blender and mix to an even paste.

Heat a pan over medium heat with a teaspoon of coconut oil and gently fry the pasta. Deglaze with coconut milk and add to the slow cooker.

Cut the zucchini into pieces, the broccoli in florets, the peppers into cubes and put in the slow cooker. Simmer for 4 hours.

Briefly heat the cauliflower rice in 1 teaspoon of coconut oil, season with a little salt and pepper in a pan over medium heat.

Nutrition:

Calories: 380 Fat: 10g Net Carbs: 44g

Fiber: 5g Protein: 30g

Chapter 3 Dinner Recipes

Thai Basil Chicken

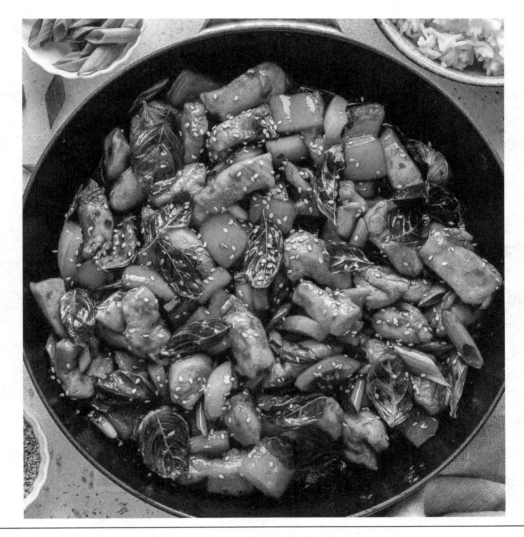

Preparation time: 10 minutes
Cooking time: 30 minutes

Servings: 1

Ingredients: For the egg:

1 egg 2 tablespoons of coconut oil for frying

Basil chicken

1 chicken breast (or any other cut of boneless chicken, about 200 grams)

5 cloves of garlic 4 Thai chilies

1 tablespoon oil for frying Fish sauce

1 handful of Thai holy basil leaves

Directions:

First, fry the egg.

Basil chicken

Cut the chicken into small pieces. Peel the garlic and chilies, and chop them fine. Add basil leaves.

Add about 1 tablespoon of oil to the pan.

When the oil is hot, add the chilies and garlic. Stir fry for half a minute.

Toss in your chicken and keep stir frying. Add fish sauce.

Add basil into the pan, fold it into the chicken, and turn off the heat.

Nutrition:

Calories: 366 Net carbs: 21g

Fat: 17.6g Fiber: 2.1g Protein: 32.2g

Shrimp with Snow Peas

Preparation time: 5 minutes
Cooking time: 10 minutes
Servings: 4.

Ingredients:

Marinade

2 teaspoons arrowroot flour

1 tablespoon red wine

½ tablespoon salt

Stir Fry

1 pound shrimp, peeled and deveined

2 tablespoon oil

1 tablespoon minced ginger

3 garlic cloves, sliced thinly

1/2 pound snow peas, strings removed

2 teaspoons fish sauce

1/4 cup chicken broth

4 green onions, white and light green parts, sliced diagonally

2 teaspoons dark roasted sesame oil

Directions:

Mix all the ingredients for the marinade in a bowl and then add the shrimp. Mix to coat. Let it marinade 15 minutes while you prepare the peas, ginger, and garlic.

Add the coconut oil in the wok and let it get hot. Add the garlic and ginger and combine. Stir-fry for about 30 seconds.

Add the marinade to the wok, add the snow peas, fish sauce and chicken broth. Stir-fry until the shrimp turns pink. Add the green onions and stir-fry for one more minute. Turn off the heat and add the sesame oil. Toss once more and serve with steamed brown rice or soba gluten free noodles.

Nutrition:

Calories: 258

Net carbs: 4.4g

Fat: 15.8g

Fiber: 0.7g

Protein: 23.5g

Cashew Chicken

Preparation time: 10 minutes
Cooking time: 10 minutes
Servings: 4

Ingredients:

1 bunch scallions

1 pound skinless boneless chicken thighs

1/2 teaspoon. Salt

1/4 teaspoon. Black pepper

1tablespoon oil

1 red bell pepper and 1 stalk of celery, chopped

4 garlic cloves, finely chopped

1 1/2 tablespoon. Finely chopped peeled fresh ginger

1/4 teaspoon. Dried hot red-pepper flakes

3/4 cup chicken broth

1 1/2 tablespoon. Fish sauce

1 1/2 teaspoons arrowroot flour

1/2 cup salted roasted whole cashews

Directions:

Chop scallions and separate green and white parts. Pat chicken dry and cut into 3/4-inch pieces and season with salt and pepper. Heat a wok or a skillet over high heat. Add oil and then stir-fry chicken until cooked through, 3 to 4 minutes. Transfer to a plate. Add garlic, bell pepper, celery, ginger, red-pepper flakes, and scallion whites to wok and stir-fry until peppers are just tender, 4 to 5 minutes.

Mix together broth, fish sauce and arrowroot flour, then stir into vegetables in wok. Reduce heat and simmer, stirring occasionally, until thickened. Stir in cashews, scallion greens, and chicken along with any juices.

Nutrition:

Calories: 264

Net carbs: 16.3g

Fat: 13.7g

Fiber: 2.6g

Protein: 19.4g

Bass Celery Tomato Bok Choy Stir Fry

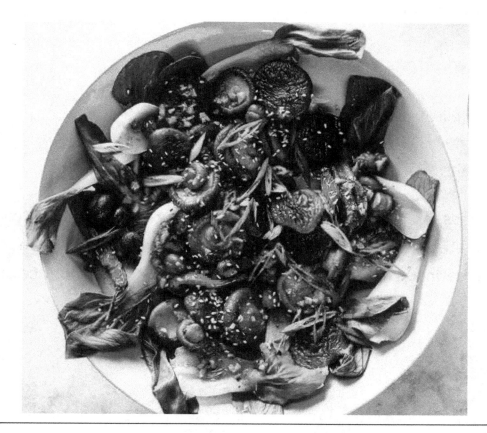

Preparation time: 5 minutes
Cooking time: 5 minutes
Servings: 2

Ingredients:

1/2 pound bass fillets

1 cup Celery

1/2 cup sliced Tomatoes

1/2 cup sliced Bok Choy

1/2 cup sliced carrots and cucumbers

1 Teaspoon oil

Directions:

Marinade bass in a Super foods marinade. Stir fry drained bass in coconut oil for few minutes, add all vegetables and stir fry for 2 more minutes. Add the rest of the marinade and stir fry for a minute. Serve with brown rice or quinoa.

Nutrition:

Calories: 152

Net carbs: 0.5g

Fat: 5.9g

Protein: 22.8g

Broccoli, Yellow Peppers & Beef Stir Fry

Preparation time: 5 minutes
Cooking time: 20 minutes
Servings: 2

Ingredients:

1/2 pound beef

1 cup Broccoli

1/2 cup sliced Yellow Peppers

1/2 cup chopped onions

1 Tablespoon. Sesame seeds

1 Teaspoon oil

Directions:

Marinade beef in a Super foods marinade. Stir fry drained beef in coconut oil for few minutes, add all vegetables and stir fry for 2 more minutes. Add the rest of the marinade and stir fry for a minute. Serve with brown rice or quinoa.

Nutrition:

Calories: 107 Net carbs: 10g

Fat: 2.1g Fiber: 5g Protein: 10g

Chinese Celery, Mushrooms & Fish Stir Fry

Preparation time: 5 minutes
Cooking time: 10 minutes
Servings: 2

Ingredients:

1/2 pound fish fillets

1 cup Chinese Celery

1 cup Mushrooms sliced in half

1/2 cup peppers sliced diagonally

1 Teaspoon oil

Directions:

Marinade fish in a Super foods marinade. Stir fry drained fish in coconut oil for few minutes, add all vegetables and stir fry for 2 more minutes. Add the rest of the marinade and stir fry for a minute. Serve with brown rice or quinoa.

Nutrition:

Calories: 24

Fat: 0.2g

Protein: 5g

Pork, Green Pepper and Tomato Stir Fry

Preparation time: 5 minutes
Cooking time: 20 minutes
Servings: 2

Ingredients:

1/2 pound cubed pork

1 cup Green Peppers

1/2 cup sliced Tomatoes

1 teaspoon. Ground black pepper

1 Teaspoon oil

Directions:

Marinade pork In a super foods marinade. Stir fry drained pork in coconut oil for few minutes, add all vegetables and stir fry for 2 more minutes. Add the rest of the marinade and stir fry for a minute. Serve with brown rice or quinoa.

Nutrition:

Calories: 86 Net carbs: 2.7g

Fat: 2.7g Fiber: 1.9g Protein: 11.6g

Pork, Red & Green Peppers, Onion & Carrots Stir Fry

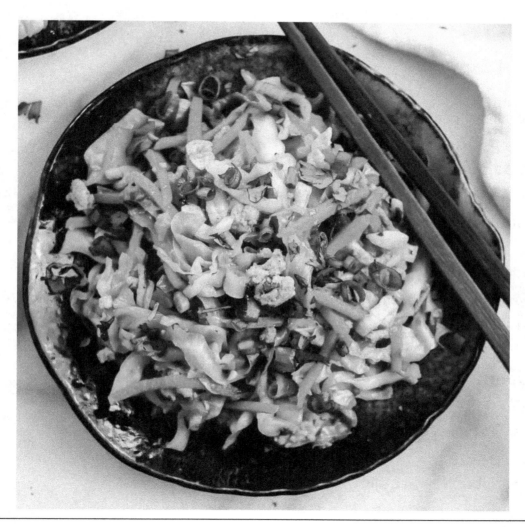

Preparation time: 5 minutes
Cooking time: 20 minutes
Servings: 2

Ingredients:

1/2 pound cubed pork

1/2 cup chopped Red Peppers

1/2 cup chopped Green Peppers

1/2 cup sliced onion

1/2 cup sliced carrots

1 Teaspoon oil

Directions:

Marinade pork in a super foods marinade. Stir fry drained pork in coconut oil for few minutes, add all vegetables and stir fry for 2 more minutes. Add the rest of the marinade and stir fry for a minute. Serve with brown rice or quinoa.

Nutrition:

Calories: 118 Net carbs: 0.7g

Fat: 2.6g Fiber: 1g Protein: 22.3g

Chicken Edamame Stir Fry

Preparation time: 5 minutes
Cooking time: 15 minutes
Servings: 2

Ingredients:

1/2 pound chicken

1 cup Edamame pre-cooked in boiling water for 3 minutes

1/2 cup sliced carrots

1 Teaspoon oil

Directions:

Marinade chicken in a super foods marinade. Stir fry drained chicken in coconut oil for few minutes, add all vegetables and stir fry for 2 more minutes. Add the rest of the marinade and stir fry for a minute. Serve with brown rice or quinoa.

Nutrition:

Calories: 295 Net carbs: 12.3g

Fat: 13.1g Protein: 31.6g

Chicken, Zucchini, Carrots and Baby Corn Stir Fry

Preparation time: 5 minutes
Cooking time: 15 minutes
Servings: 2

Ingredients:

1/2 pound chicken

1 cup Zucchini

1/2 cup sliced Carrots

1/2 cup Baby Corn

1 Tablespoon. Chopped Cilantro

1 Teaspoon oil

Directions:

Marinade chicken in a super foods marinade. Stir fry drained chicken in coconut oil for few minutes, add all vegetables and stir fry for 2 more minutes. Add the rest of the marinade and stir fry for a minute. Serve with brown rice or quinoa over bed of lettuce.

Nutrition:

Calories: 187 Net carbs: 7.4g Fat: 6g

Fiber: 5.7g Protein: 26.2g

Vegan Stir Fry

Preparation time: 5 minutes
Cooking time: 5 minutes
Servings: 2

Ingredients:

1/2 pound shiitake mushrooms

1/2 cup Chinese Celery

1/2 cup sliced carrots and cucumbers

1 Teaspoon oil

Directions:

Marinade mushrooms in a super foods marinade. Stir fry drained mushrooms in coconut oil for few minutes, add all other vegetables and stir fry for 2 more minutes. Add the rest of the marinade and stir fry for a minute. Serve with brown rice or quinoa.

Nutrition:

Calories: 122 Net carbs: 8.7g Fat: 6.9g

Fiber: 1.7g Protein:7.3g

Eggplant, Chinese Celery & Peppers Stir Fry

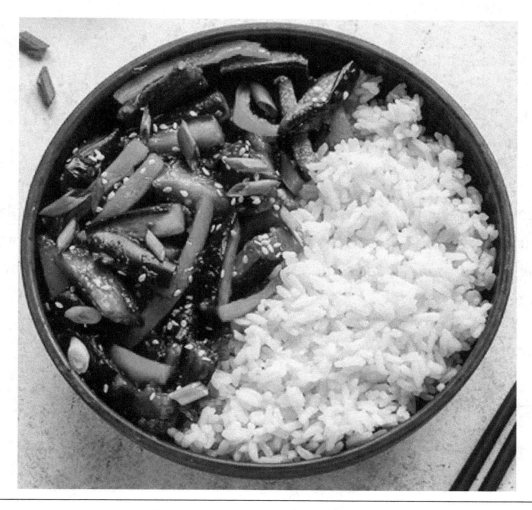

Preparation time: 5 minutes
Cooking time: 5 minutes
Servings: 2

Ingredients:

1/2 pound cubed eggplant

1/2 cup Chinese Celery

1/2 cup sliced Red Peppers

1/4 cup sliced chili Peppers

1 Teaspoon. Oil

Directions:

Marinade eggplant in a super foods marinade. Stir fry drained eggplant in coconut oil for few minutes, add all vegetables and stir fry for 2 more minutes. Add the rest of the marinade and stir fry for a minute. Serve with brown rice or quinoa.

Nutrition:

Calories: 14 Net carbs: 2.1g

Fat: 0.1g Fiber: 1g Protein: 0.9

Pork Fried Brown Rice

Preparation time: 5 minutes
Cooking time: 35 minutes
Servings: 2

Ingredients:

1/2 pound cubed pork

1 cup Peppers

1/2 cup sliced Carrots

1 Tablespoon. Black sesame seeds

1 cup cooked brown rice

1 Teaspoon oil

Directions:

Marinade pork in a super foods marinade. Stir fry drained pork in coconut oil for few minutes, add all vegetables and stir fry for 2 more minutes. Add the rest of the marinade and stir fry for a minute. Stir in brown rice and black sesame seeds.

Nutrition:

Calories: 335 Net carbs: 41.9g Fat: 12.8g

Fiber: 1.4g Protein: 11.9g

Chicken, Red Peppers, Zucchini & Cashews Stir Fry

Preparation time: 5 minutes
Cooking time: 15 minutes
Servings: 2

Ingredients:

1/2 pound chicken

1 cup Zucchini

1/2 cup sliced Red Peppers

1/2 cup sliced scallions

1/4 cup Cashews

1 Teaspoon. Oil

Directions:

Marinade chicken in a super foods marinade. Stir fry drained chicken in coconut oil for few minutes, add all vegetables and stir fry for 2 more minutes. Add the rest of the marinade and stir fry for a minute. Serve with brown rice or quinoa.

Nutrition:

Calories: 295

Net carbs: 12.3g

Fat: 13.1g

Protein: 31.6g

Chapter 4 Snacks

Apple Pastry

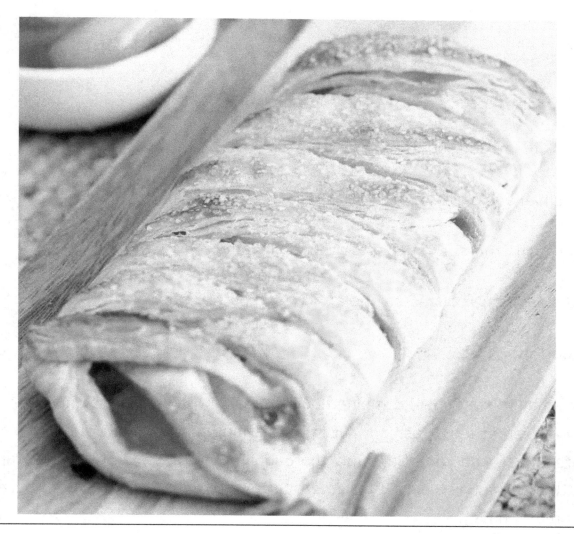

Preparation time: 15 minutes
Cooking time: 30 minutes

Servings: 1

Ingredients:

Three cups all-purpose flour

Dash of salt

Two teaspoons margarine

One plain low-fat yogurt

One small apple

Dash each ground nutmeg and ground cinnamon

Two teaspoons reduced-calorie apricot spread (16 calories per 2 teaspoons)

Directions:

In a small mixing bowl, combine flour and salt; with a pastry blender, or two knives used scissors-fashion, cut in margarine until the mixture resembles a coarse meal. Add yogurt and mix thoroughly. Form dough into a ball; wrap in plastic wrap and refrigerate for at least 1 hour (maybe kept in the refrigerator for up to 3 days).

Between 2 sheets of a wax paper roll dough, forming a 4/2-inch circle about 1/2. Inch thick. Carefully remove wax paper and place dough on foil or small cookie sheet—Preheat oven to 350°F.

Core, pare, and thinly slice apple; arrange slices decoratively over the dough and sprinkle with nutmeg and cinnamon. Bake until crust is golden, 20 to 30 minutes.

During the last few minutes, that pastry is baking, in a small metal measuring cup or other small flameproof container heat apricot spread; as soon as the pie is done, brush with a warm space.

Nutrition:

238 calories;

4 g protein;

8 g fat;

38 g carbohydrate;

228 mg sodium;

1 mg cholesterol.

Baked Maple Apple

Preparation time: 10 minutes
Cooking time: 30 minutes
Servings: 2

Ingredients:

Two small apples

Two teaspoons reduced-calorie apricot

Spread

One teaspoon reduced-calorie maple-flavored syrup

Directions:

Remove the core from each apple to 1/2 inch from the bottom. Remove a thin strip of peel from around the center of each apple (this helps keep skin from bursting). Fill each apple with one teaspoon apricot spread and 1/2 teaspoon maple syrup. Place each apple upright in individual baking dish; cover dishes with foil and bake at 400°F until apples are tender, 25 to 30 minutes.

Nutrition:

75 calories; 0.2 g protein; 1 g fat;

19 g carbohydrate; 0.3 mg sodium;

Apple-Raisin Cake

Preparation time: 20 minutes
Cooking time: 50 minutes
Servings: 12

Ingredients: One teaspoon baking soda

1/2 cups applesauce (no sugar added)

Two small Golden Delicious apples, cored, pared, and shredded

1 cup less 2 s raisins

2/4 cups self-rising flour

1 teaspoon ground cinnamon

1/2 teaspoon ground cloves 1/3 cup plus 2 teaspoons unsalted margarine

1/4 cup granulated sugar

Directions:

Spray an 8 x 8 x 2-inch baking pan with nonstick cooking spray and set aside. Into a medium bowl sift together flour, cinnamon, and cloves; set aside.Preheat oven to 350°F. In a medium mixing bowl, using an electric mixer, cream margarine, add sugar and stir to combine. Stir baking soda into applesauce, then add to margarine mixture and stir to combine; add sifted ingredients and, using an electric mixer on medium speed, beat until thoroughly combined. Fold in apples and raisins; pour batter into the sprayed pan and bake for 45 to 50 minutes (until cake is browned and a cake tester or toothpick, inserted in center, comes out dry). Remove cake from pan and cool on wire rack.

Nutrition: 151 calories; 2 g protein;

4 g fat; 28 g carbohydrate; 96 mg sodium;

Cinnamon-Apricot Bananas

Preparation time: 45 minutes
Cooking time: 0 minutes
Servings: 2

Ingredients:

4 graham crackers 2x2-inch 1 medium banana, peeled and cut in squares), made into crumbs half lengthwise

2 teaspoons shredded coconut

1/4 teaspoon ground cinnamon

1 plus 1 teaspoon reduced-calorie apricot spread (16 calories per 2 teaspoons)

Directions:

In small skillet combine crumbs, coconut, and cinnamon and toast lightly, being careful not to burn; transfer to a sheet of wax paper or a paper plate and set aside.

In the same skillet heat apricot spread until melted; remove from heat. Roll each banana half in a spread, then quickly roll in crumb mixture, pressing crumbs so that they adhere to the banana; place coated halves on a plate, cover lightly, and refrigerate until chilled.

Variation: Coconut-Strawberry Bananas —Omit cinnamon and substitute reduced-calorie strawberry spread (16 calories per 2 teaspoons) for the apricot spread.

Nutrition:

130 calories; 2g protein;

2g fat; 29g carbohydrate;

95mg sodium;

Meringue Crepes with Blueberry Custard Filling

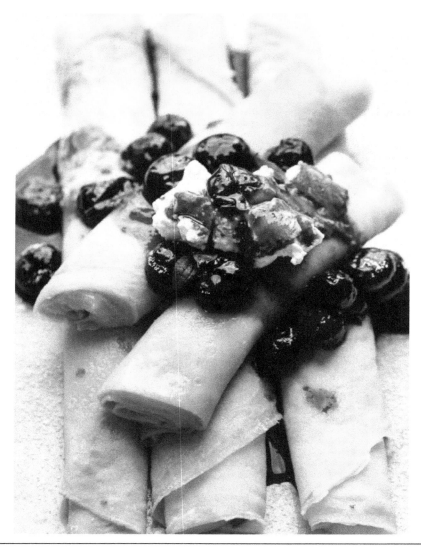

Preparation time: 10 minutes
Cooking time: 20 minutes
Servings: 4

Ingredients:

2 cups blueberries (reserve 8 berries for garnish)

1 cup evaporated skimmed milk

2 large eggs, separated

1 plus 1 teaspoon granulated sugar, divided

2 teaspoons each cornstarch

Lemon juice

Directions:

In 1-quart saucepan, combine milk, egg yolks, and one sugar; cook over low heat, continually stirring, until slightly thickened and bubbles form around sides of the mixture. In a cup or small bowl dissolve cornstarch in lemon juice; gradually stir into milk mixture and cook, constantly stirring, until thick. Remove from heat and fold in blueberries; let cool.

Spoon Vs. of custard onto the center of each crepe and fold sides over filling to enclose; arrange crepes, seam-side down, in an 8 x 8 x 2-inch baking pan. In a small bowl, using an electric mixer on high speed, beat egg whites until soft peaks form; add remaining teaspoon sugar, and continue beating until stiff peaks form.

Fill the pastry bag with egg whites and pipe an equal amount over each crepe (if pastry bag is not available, spoon egg whites over crepes); top each with a reserved blueberry and broil until meringue is lightly browned, 10 to 15 seconds. Serve immediately.

Nutrition:

300 calories;

16g protein;

6g fat;

45g carbohydrate;

180mg sodium;

278mg cholesterol

Chilled Cherry Soup

Preparation time: 5 minutes
Cooking time: 5 minutes
Servings: 2

Ingredients:

20 large frozen pitted cherries (no sugar added)

1/2 cup water

1/2 teaspoons granulated sugar

2-inch cinnamon stick

1 strip lemon peel

2 s rose wine

1 teaspoon cornstarch

1/4 cup plain low-fat yogurt

Directions:

In a small saucepan, combine cherries, water, sugar, cinnamon stick, and lemon peel; bring to a boil. Reduce heat, cover, and let simmer for 20 minutes.

Remove and discard the cinnamon stick and lemon peel from a cherry mixture. In measuring cup or small bowl combine wine and cornstarch, stirring to dissolve cornstarch; add to cherry mixture and, constantly stirring, bring to a boil. Reduce heat and let simmer until the mixture thickens.

In a heatproof bowl, stir yogurt until smooth; add cherry mixture and stir to combine. Cover with plastic wrap and refrigerate until well chilled

Nutrition:

98 calories;

2 g protein;

1 g fat;

19 g carbohydrate;

21 mg sodium;

2 mg cholesterol

Iced Orange Punch

Preparation time: 20 minutes
Cooking time: 0 minutes
Servings: 8

Ingredients:

Ice Mold Club soda

1 lemon, sliced 1 lime, sliced

Punch

1 quart each chilled orange juice (no sugar added), club soda, and diet ginger ale)

Directions:

To Prepare Ice Mold: Pour enough club soda into a 10- or 12-cup ring mold to fill mold; add lemon and lime slices, arranging them in an alternating pattern. Cover the mold and carefully transfer to freezer; freeze until solid.

To Prepare Punch: In a large punch bowl, combine juice and sodas. Remove ice mold from ring mold and float ice mold in a punch.

Nutrition:

56 calories; 1g protein; 0.1 g fat;

14 g carbohydrate; 35 mg sodium;

Meatless Borscht

Preparation time: 15 minutes
Cooking time: 45 minutes
Servings: 2

Ingredients: 1 teaspoon margarine

1 cup shredded green cabbage

1/4 cup chopped onion

1/4 cup sliced carrot

1 cup coarsely shredded pared

2 s tomato paste beets 1 lemon juice

2 cups of water

1/2 teaspoon granulated sugar

2 packets instant beef broth and 1 teaspoon pepper

Seasoning mix 1/2 bay leaf

1/4 cup plain low-fat yogurt

Directions: In 1 1/2-quart saucepan heat margarine until bubbly and hot; add onion and sauté until softened, 1 to 2 minutes. Add beets and toss to combine; add water, broth mix, and bay leaf and bring to a boil. Cover pan and cook over medium heat for 10 minutes; stir in remaining ingredients except for yogurt, cover, and let simmer until vegetables are tender about 25 minutes. Remove and discard bay leaf. Pour borscht into 2 soup bowls and top each portion with 2 s yogurt.

Nutrition: 120 calories; 5g protein; 3g fat;

21g carbohydrate; 982mg sodium;

2mg cholesterol

Sautéed Sweet 'N' Sour Beets

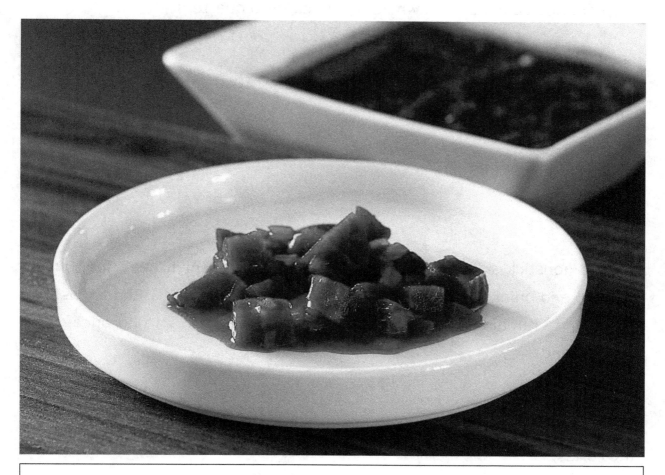

Preparation time: 10 minutes
Cooking time: 10 minutes
Servings: 2

Ingredients:

Serve hot or chilled.

2 teaspoons margarine

1 diced onion

1 cup drained canned small whole beets, cut into quarters

1 each lemon juice and water

1 teaspoon each salt and pepper

Dash granulated sugar substitute

Directions:

In small nonstick skillet heat margarine over medium-high heat until bubbly and hot; add onion and sauté until softened, 1 to 2 minutes. Reduce heat to low and add remaining ingredients; cover pan and cook, stirring once, for 5 minutes longer.

Nutrition:

70 calories;

1g protein;

4g fat;

9g carbohydrate;

385 mg sodium;

Orange Beets

Preparation time: 10 minutes
Cooking time: 10 minutes
Servings: 2

Ingredients:

1 /2 teaspoons lemon juice

1 teaspoon cornstarch Dash salt

1 teaspoon orange marmalade

1 cup peeled and sliced cooked beets

2 teaspoons margarine

1 teaspoon firmly packed brown

Sugar 1/4 cup orange juice (no sugar added)

Directions:

In a 1-quart saucepan (not aluminum or cast-iron), combine beets, margarine, and sugar; cook over low heat, continually stirring until margarine and sugar are melted.

In 1-cup measure or small bowl combine juices, cornstarch, and salt, stirring to dissolve cornstarch; pour over beet mixture and, constantly stirring, bring to a boil. Continue cooking and stirring

Until the mixture thickens.

Reduce heat, add marmalade, and stir until combined. Remove from heat and let cool slightly; cover and refrigerate for at least 1 hour. Reheat before serving.

Nutrition:

99 calories; 1g protein; 4g fat;

16g carbohydrate; 146mg sodium;

Cabbage 'N' Potato Soup

Preparation time: 10 minutes
Cooking time: 40 minutes
Servings: 4

Ingredients:

This soup freezes well; for easy portion control, freeze in pre-measured servings.

2 teaspoons vegetable oil

4 cups shredded green cabbage

1 cup sliced onions

1 garlic clove, minced

3 cups of water

6 ounces peeled potato, sliced

1 cup each sliced carrot and tomato puree

4 packets instant beef broth and seasoning mix

1 each bay leaf and whole clove

Directions:

In 2-quart saucepan heat oil, add cabbage, onions, and garlic and sauté over medium heat, frequently stirring, until cabbage is soft, about 10 minutes. Reduce heat to low and add remaining ingredients; cook until vegetables are tender, about 30 minutes. Remove and discard bay leaf and clove before serving.

Nutrition:

119 calories; 4 g protein; 3 g fat;

22 g carbohydrate; 900 mg sodium,

Eggplant Pesto

Preparation time: 15 minutes
Cooking time: 30 minutes
Servings: 2

Ingredients:

1 medium eggplant (about 1 pound), cut crosswise into thick rounds

Dash salt

Fresh basil and grated Parmesan cheese

1 olive oil

1 small garlic clove, mashed

Dash freshly ground pepper

Directions:

On 10 X 15-inch nonstick baking sheet arrange eggplant slices in a single layer; sprinkle with salt and bake at 425°F. Until easily pierced with a fork, about 30 minutes.

In a small bowl, combine remaining ingredients; spread an equal amount of mixture over each eggplant slice. Transfer slices to I1/2-quart casserole, return to oven, and bake until heated, about 10 minutes longer.

Nutrition:

144 calories;

5g protein;

9g fat;

14g carbohydrate;

163mg sodium;

4mg cholesterol

Chapter 5 Desserts Recipes

Raw Vegan Carrot Cake

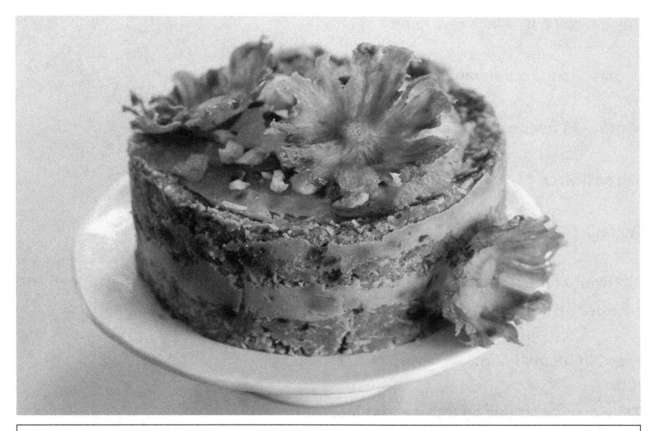

Preparation time: 10 minutes
Cooking time: 35 minutes
Servings: 4

Ingredients: Crust:

4 carrots, chopped 1½ cups oats

½ cup dried coconut 2 cups dates

1 teaspoon cinnamon ½ teaspoon nutmeg

1½ cups cashews 2 coconut oil

Juice from 1 lemon 2 raw honey

1 teaspoon ground vanilla bean

Water, as needed

Directions:

Add all crust ingredients to the blender.

Mix well and optionally add a couple of drops of water at a time to make the mixture stick together.

Press in a small pan.

Take it out and put on a plate and freeze.

Mix frosting ingredients in a blender and add water if necessary.

Add frosting to the crust and refrigerate.

Nutrition:

Calories: 241 Net carbs: 28.4g

Fat: 13.4g Fiber: 0.8g Protein: 2.4g

Frozen Raw Blackberry Cake

Preparation time: 10 minutes
Cooking time: 45 minutes
Servings: 4

Ingredients: Crust:

3/4 cup shredded coconut

15 dried dates soaked in hot water and drained

1/3 cup pumpkin seeds 1/4 cup of coconut oil

Middle filling Coconut whipped cream

Top filling:

1 pound of frozen blackberries

3-4 raw honey 1/4 cup of coconut cream

2 egg whites

Directions:

Grease the cake tin with coconut oil and mix all base ingredients in the blender until you get a sticky ball. Press the base mixture in a cake tin. Freeze. Make

Coconut Whipped Cream. Process berries and add honey, coconut cream and egg whites. Pour middle filling - Coconut Whipped Cream in the tin and spread evenly. Freeze. Pour top filling - berries mixture-in the tin, spread, decorate with blueberries and almonds and return to freezer.

Nutrition:

Calories: 472 Net carbs: 15.8g Fat: 18g

Fiber: 16.8g Protein: 33.3g

Chocolate Chip Gelato

Preparation time: 30 minutes
Cooking time: 0 minutes
Servings: 4

Ingredients:

2 cups dairy-free milk

¾ cup pure maple syrup

1 pure vanilla extract

⅓ Semi-sweet vegan chocolate chips, finely chopped or flaked

Directions:

Beat dairy-free milk, maple syrup, and vanilla together in a large bowl until well combined.

Pour the mixture carefully into the container of an automatic ice cream maker and process it according to the manufacturer's instructions.

During the last 10 or 15 minutes, add the chopped chocolate and continue processing until the desired texture is achieved. Enjoy the gelato immediately, or let it harden further in the freezer for an hour or more.

Nutrition:

Calories: 94

Net carbs: 14.9g

Fat: 3.4g

Fiber: 0.5g

Protein: 0.8g

Peanut Butter And Jelly Ice Cream

Preparation time: 40 minutes
Cooking time: 0 minutes
Servings: 6

Ingredients:

2 cups dairy-free milk, simple, sugar-free

⅔ Cup maple syrup

3 s creamy natural peanut butter

½ teaspoon ground ginger

2 teaspoons pure vanilla extract

6 spoons canned fruits

Directions:

Beat the milk without milk, maple syrup, peanut butter, and vanilla in a large bowl until well combined. Pour the mixture carefully into the container of an automatic ice cream maker and process it according to the manufacturer's instructions.

Add canned fruits for the last 10 minutes, and let them combine with the ice cream until the desired texture is achieved. Enjoy the ice cream immediately, or let it harden further in the freezer for an hour or more.

Nutrition: Calories: 189 Net carbs: 33.8g

Fat: 4.1g Fiber: 0.7g Protein: 5.6g

Watermelon Gazpacho In A Jar

Preparation time: 20 minutes
Cooking time: 0 minutes
Servings: 8

Ingredients:

1kg of ripe, aromatic tomatoes

Half a red pepper +

Half a small chili pepper

3 ground cucumbers

1 onion

1 clove of garlic (optional)

2 cups cubed watermelon

Juice of 1 lemon

A handful of leaves basil

A handful of mint leaves

1 - 2 s olive oil

Salt, pepper

Directions:

Tomato peel slightly cut in several places, then transfer the tomatoes to a deep pot and pour boiling water, let stand for a few minutes. Drain the water and peel the tomatoes from the skin, but this is not a necessary stage if the skin does not bother you.

Peeled tomatoes in half and put in a blender cup or larger bowl. Add chopped onion, garlic, diced peppers, cucumbers, chili peppers, and lemon juice. Also, add basil and mint leaves. All mix well in a blender or using a hand blender, finally adding olive oil.

Then add chopped pieces of watermelon and mix only for a moment, so that the remaining watermelon particles can be felt. Season with salt and pepper to taste.

Serve well chilled with diced paprika, lemon juice, stale bread, and a large dose of fresh, chopped basil.

Nutrition:

Calories: 46

Net carbs: 4.3g

Fat: 0.2g

Fiber: 0.5g

Protein: 7g

Raw Vegan Chocolate Hazelnuts Truffles

Preparation time: 10 minutes
Cooking time: 30 minutes
Servings: 4

Ingredients:

1 cup ground almonds

1 teaspoon ground vanilla bean

½ cup of coconut oil

½ cup mashed pitted dates

12 whole hazelnuts

2 cacao powder

Directions:

Mix all ingredients and make truffles with one whole hazelnut in the middle.

Nutrition:

Calories: 370

Net carbs: 66.9g

Fat: 11.8g

Fiber: 2.6g

Protein: 4.2g

Raw Vegan Chocolate Cream Fruity Cake

Preparation time: 10 minutes
Cooking time: 45 minutes
Servings: 4

Ingredients:

Chocolate cream: 1 avocado

2 raw honey 2 coconut oil

2 cacao powder

1 teaspoon ground vanilla bean

Pinch of sea salt

¼ cup of coconut milk

1 coconut flakes

Fruits:

1 chopped banana

1 cup pitted cherries

Directions:

Prepare the crust and press it at the bottom of the pan.

Blend all chocolate cream ingredients, fold in the fruits and pour in the crust.

Whip the top layer, spread and sprinkle with cacao powder.

Refrigerate.

Nutrition:

Calories: 106 Net carbs: 0.4g Fat: 5g

Fiber: 0.1g Protein: 14g

Jerusalem Artichoke Gratin

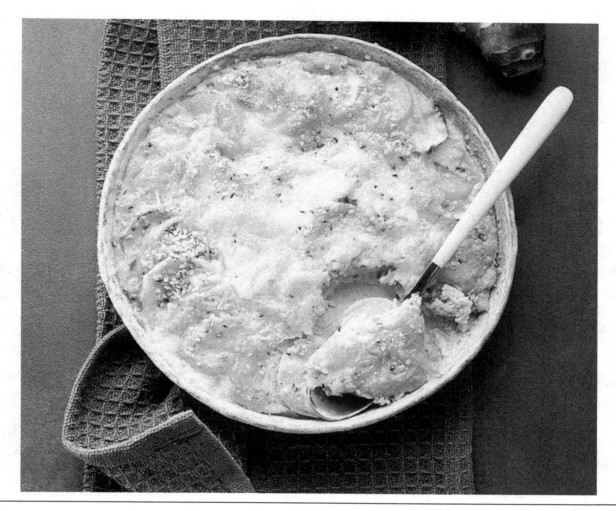

Preparation time: 10 minutes
Cooking time: 45 minutes
Servings: 3

Ingredients:

600g Jerusalem artichoke

250ml of milk

2 grated cheese

1 crème fraiche

1 butter

Curry, paprika powder, nutmeg, salt, pepper

Directions:

Wash and peel the Jerusalem artichoke tubers and slice them into approx. 3 mm thick slices. Bring them to a boil with the milk in a saucepan. Then stir in the spices and crème fraiche.

Grease a baking dish with butter and add the Jerusalem artichoke and milk mixture. Bake on the middle shelf in the oven for about half an hour at 160 ° C. Sprinkle with grated cheese and bake five minutes before the end of the baking time. Gorgeous!

Nutrition:

Calories: 133

Net carbs: 9.9g

Fat: 8.1g

Fiber: 1.1g

Protein: 4.7g

Baked Quinces With A Cream Crown

Preparation time: 20 minutes
Cooking time: 90 minutes
Servings: 1

Ingredients:

1-2 quinces

70-80 g whipped cream

1 teaspoon sugar

1 teaspoon vanilla sugar

Directions:

After you have freed the quince from its fluff, you wrap it loosely in aluminum foil and put it in the oven at 200 ° C for 60 to 90 minutes, the thicker the fruit, the longer the baking time.

Spend the wait waiting to whip the cream stiff and sweeten it.

When the quinces have softened, halve them, remove the core with a small spoon and then pour the sweet whipped cream into this trough.

Nutrition:

Calories: 52

Net carbs: 14g

Fiber: 1.7g

Protein: 0.3g

Apple And Pear Jam With Tarragon

Preparation time: 15 minutes
Cooking time: 0 minutes
Servings: 3

Ingredients:

500g juicy pears

500g sour apples

1 large lemon

2 sprigs of tarragon

500g jam sugar 2: 1

Directions:

Peel and quarter apples and pears, remove the core and dice or grate very, very finely.

Squeeze the lemon and add to the fruit with the gelling sugar.

Let the juice soak overnight!

Wash and dry the tarragon. Finely chop the leaves and add to the fruit mix.

Nutrition:

Calories: 242

Net carbs: 15g

Fat: 20.5g

Fiber: 3.2g

Protein: 2g

Apple Jam With Honey And Cinnamon

Preparation time: 10 minutes
Cooking time: 15 minutes
Servings: 2

Ingredients:

300g apples

6 lemon juice

2 sticks of cinnamon

50 g liquid honey,

500g jam sugar 2: 1

Directions:

Peel and quarter the apples and remove the core.

Weigh 1 kg of pulp. Dice this finely and drizzle with lemon juice.

Mix the pulp, gelling sugar and cinnamon sticks well in a large saucepan.

After cooking remove the cinnamon sticks and stir in the honey.

Nutrition:

Calories: 193 Net carbs: 38g Fat: 4.5g

Fiber: 1.8g Protein: 1.8g

Plum Chutney

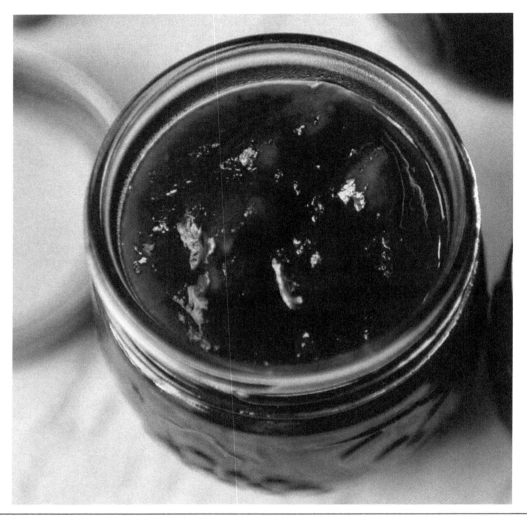

Preparation time: 5 minutes
Cooking time: 50 minutes
Servings: 4

Ingredients:

500 g pitted prunes

50 g ginger

350 g onions

2 s vegetable oil

250g brown sugar

300ml balsamic vinegar

Salt, pepper

Directions:

Quarter the washed and pitted plums. Finely dice the ginger and onions and braise in 2 s of oil. Add the plums and steam briefly.

Add the brown sugar and let it melt while stirring. Then pour balsamic vinegar over it and let it boil for about 40 minutes on a low flame.

Season with salt and pepper and pour into boiled glasses.

Nutrition:

Calories: 125

Net carbs: 19.6g

Fat: 4.9g

Fiber: 0.8g

Protein: 1.7g

Chocolate Chip Gelato

Preparation time: 30 minutes
Cooking time: 0 minutes
Servings: 4

Ingredients:

2 cups dairy-free milk

¾ cup pure maple syrup

1 pure vanilla extract

⅓ Semi-sweet vegan chocolate chips, finely chopped or flaked

Directions:

Beat dairy-free milk, maple syrup, and vanilla together in a large bowl until well combined.

Pour the mixture carefully into the container of an automatic ice cream maker and process it according to the manufacturer's instructions.

During the last 10 or 15 minutes, add the chopped chocolate and continue processing until the desired texture is achieved. Enjoy the gelato immediately, or let it harden further in the freezer for an hour or more.

Nutrition:

Calories: 94

Net carbs: 14.9g

Fat: 3.4g

Fiber: 0.5g

Protein: 0.8g

Peanut Butter And Jelly Ice Cream

Preparation time: 40 minutes
Cooking time: 0 minutes
Servings: 6

Ingredients:

2 cups dairy-free milk, simple, sugar-free

⅔ Cup maple syrup

3 s creamy natural peanut butter

½ teaspoon ground ginger

2 teaspoons pure vanilla extract

6 spoons canned fruits

Directions:

Beat the milk without milk, maple syrup, peanut butter, and vanilla in a large bowl until well combined. Pour the mixture carefully into the container of an automatic ice cream maker and process it according to the manufacturer's instructions.

Add canned fruits for the last 10 minutes, and let them combine with the ice cream until the desired texture is achieved. Enjoy the ice cream immediately, or let it harden further in the freezer for an hour or more.

Nutrition: Calories: 189 Net carbs: 33.8g

Fat: 4.1g Fiber: 0.7g Protein: 5.6g

Watermelon Gazpacho In A Jar

Preparation time: 20 minutes
Cooking time: 0 minutes
Servings: 8

Ingredients:

1kg of ripe, aromatic tomatoes

Half a red pepper +

Half a small chili pepper

3 ground cucumbers

1 onion

1 clove of garlic (optional)

2 cups cubed watermelon

Juice of 1 lemon

A handful of leaves basil

A handful of mint leaves

1 - 2 s olive oil

Salt, pepper

Directions:

Tomato peel slightly cut in several places, then transfer the tomatoes to a deep pot and pour boiling water, let stand for a few minutes. Drain the water and peel the tomatoes from the skin, but this is not a necessary stage if the skin does not bother you.

Peeled tomatoes in half and put in a blender cup or larger bowl. Add chopped onion, garlic, diced peppers, cucumbers, chili peppers, and lemon juice. Also, add basil and mint leaves. All mix well in a blender or using a hand blender, finally adding olive oil.

Then add chopped pieces of watermelon and mix only for a moment, so that the remaining watermelon particles can be felt. Season with salt and pepper to taste.

Serve well chilled with diced paprika, lemon juice, stale bread, and a large dose of fresh, chopped basil.

Nutrition:

Calories: 46

Net carbs: 4.3g

Fat: 0.2g

Fiber: 0.5g

Protein: 7g

Conclusion

I wish you taken pleasure in guide; thanks for making it this much.

Attempt the dishes numerous times for finest outcomes, do not neglect to speak with a physician as well as consume mindfully. Never ever quit to read more regarding your body and also constantly attempt to treat it much better.

Joy is at hand, maintain on your own healthy and balanced as well as real-time fantastic.

See you quickly with even more wonderful dishes.

CPSIA information can be obtained
at www.ICGtesting.com
Printed in the USA
LVHW060220240421
685369LV00014B/463